August 2019

HOPE

Brain Injury
HOPE
MAGAZINE
"Supporting the
Brain Injury Community"

Welcome

HOPE MAGAZINE

Serving the Brain Injury Community

August 2019

Publisher
David A. Grant

Editor
Sarah Grant

Our Contributors

Christopher Jay
Carmen Kumm
Ventura Manzanares
Bode & Debbie McKay
Jackie Otto
Ted Stachulski
Cole Taylor
Barbara Webster

Welcome to the August 2019 issue of HOPE Magazine

In this issue, we have perhaps some of the most raw and real stories submitted by our contributing writers. I am humbled by the courage these souls showed by putting their stories out there to help others.

There are not always happy endings. But endings can come in ways unexpected and serve a greater good.

The common thread with all the survivors we are featuring in this month's issue is this: They survived and are moving forward living lives of purpose as best they can.

The deeper the abyss, the greater the glory in climbing out of it.

I hope you enjoy this month's issue of HOPE Magazine!

David A. Grant
Publisher

Contents

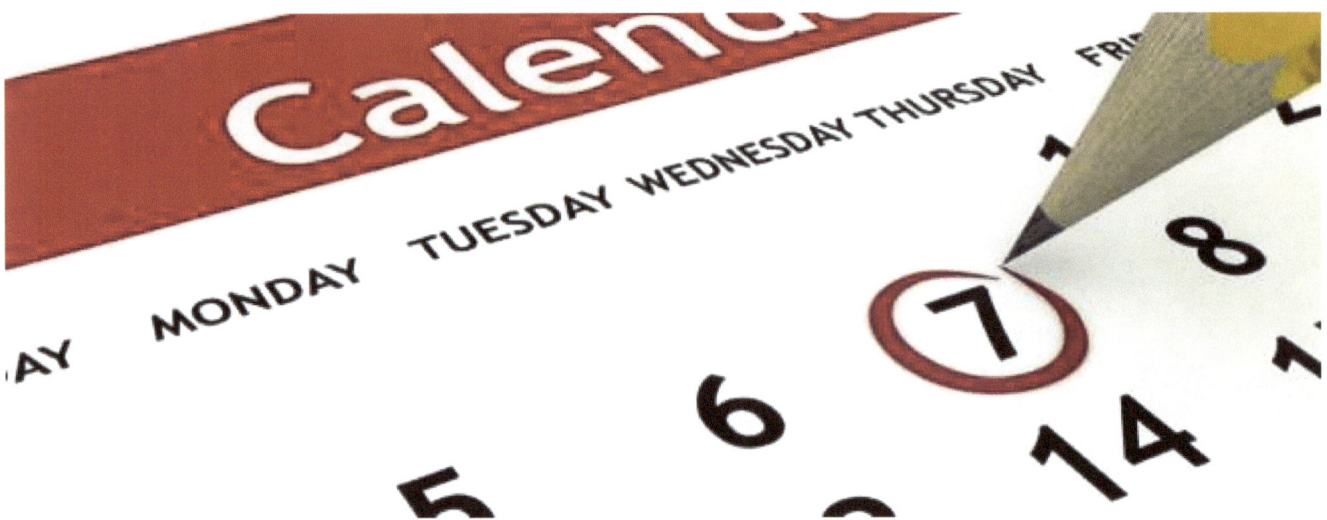

The Day That Changed Everything

By Jackie Otto

It was February 10, 2011, and it was the day that changed everything.

It was 10:00 AM. I was at work at the public school district where I have worked for the past nineteen years. At the time, I was an LRS (Learning Resource Specialist) and had thirteen schools in my zone. I worked with those schools and helped teachers with classroom management, students' behavior, and anything else that was requested by any of them.

I have had a lot of experience with behavior over my twenty-five years in education. Somehow, my life always seems to cycle back to behavior.

> "Somehow, my life always seems to cycle back to behavior."

Anything having to do with behavior is actually my love, and I would have no idea how much I would need all of that training on such a personal level.

I was at one of my schools and in a former colleague's office catching up on her life for a moment before I started my day, when my cell phone rang. It was the school where my office was located, and the gal said that a police officer had been trying to get ahold of me to tell me there had been an accident. After I hung up, all I could think of was, "An accident? A car accident? What kind of accident?"

My world stopped as my friend tried to console me and help me figure out what to do next. I decided to call the sheriff's office and try to track down the officer that way. As soon as I dialed, my phone rang again. This time it was the police officer who had been trying to find me. He said my husband had fallen off of our roof at home, and that his prognosis was not good.

My mind raced. Is this the way they tell you your husband didn't make it until you get there in person? My friend grabbed her purse and without another word said, "Where are we going?" Lee Memorial Hospital was my answer. I did have some feeling of relief knowing that it is one of the best trauma centers in the state of Florida.

That car ride was a complete blur to me, and I'm not sure what the conversation was. I do remember not being able to get there fast enough. I was also terrified of walking in – not sure of what I would find.

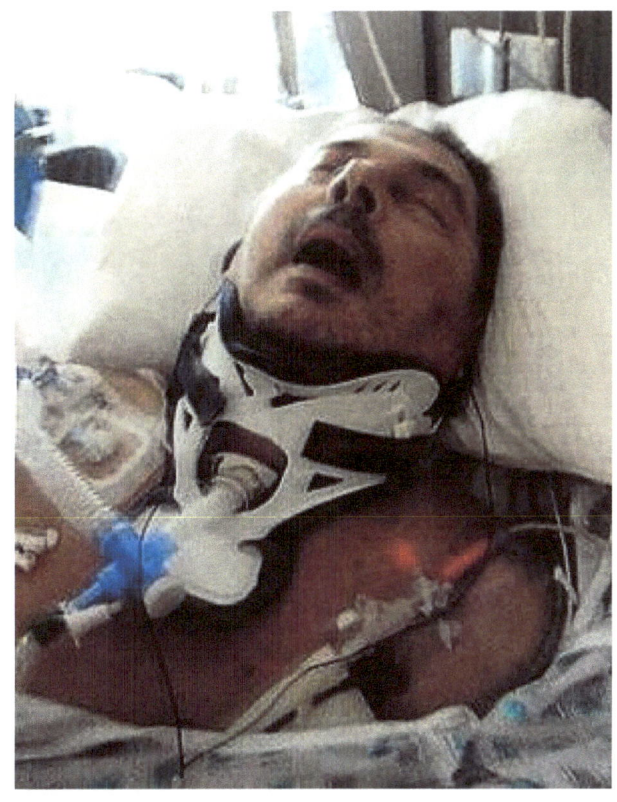

Mark – Post Surgery

Being left with your own thoughts during times of crisis is terrifying.

Once we finally arrived, the doors opened into the ER and I announced who I was to the lady behind the window. She told me to have a seat. Have a seat? Did she know what had happened to my husband?

I hardly made it to a chair when I heard my name being called. Another friend, who was an Assistant Principal at the time, met us at the hospital. I remember they both stood at my side as Kathy, the social worker, reeled off the long list of injuries that my husband had sustained during his fall off of our roof.

Broken back, broken neck, punctured lung, broken clavicle, fractured wrist, fractured ribs, and a TBI (traumatic brain injury), along with a literal brain shift. With a broken back and broken neck, I wondered if he was paralyzed. Thankfully, he was not.

I did not realize at the time that his brain bleed was the biggest concern.

I went to see him and walked right by him lying on a gurney. At that time, after twenty years together, I didn't even recognize his swollen face, head, body and the many attached machines that were now part of my husband.

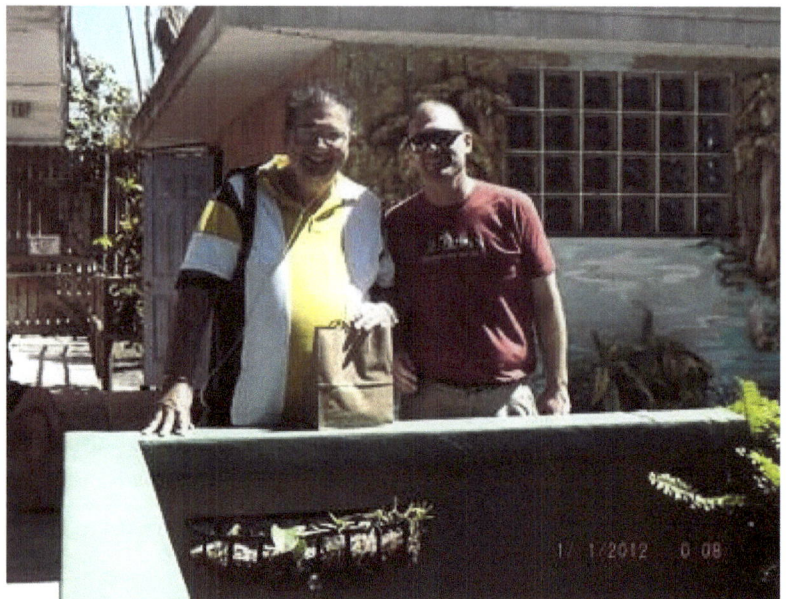
Mark and His Son Justin – Taken Last Year

The trauma doctor said, "We've got to go to surgery - now!" I watched as they wheeled my husband right by me and out of the ER. He was being kept alive by machines.

My mind was so vacant, and the pessimistic thoughts would not stop. My world had come to a dead standstill for the moment, as well as the next three hours while he underwent emergency surgery for his brain bleed. That meant he would have a craniotomy where they took a bone flap out to allow room for his damaged brain to swell.

I could not, and would not, stand and pace the floor for the next three hours. I would be next in surgery if I had to stay there while left to my own thoughts. I called my sister-in-law. She is always calm and rational. I told her what had happened to her brother. She said she would pack and be on her way. In the meantime, I went back to Lehigh to retrieve my car.

It is about a three-and-a-half hour drive from Homestead to Fort Myers by car, so I had some time to waste. One of my neighbors came running down the street when she saw me and asked if she could help. I asked her to ride back to the hospital with me. She jumped in, and off we went. The only thing I picked up was my cell phone charger. It would later prove to be my lifeline.

Once my sister-in-law got there, I felt like I would be safe, and she could help me stay calm and help me understand what the doctors were saying. It is so easy to misunderstand things when your emotional state is heightened.

It was a long three days while we had to wait and see what happened next. They told us that he was headed in the right direction.

Mark's son Justin flew in from New Hampshire, but I have no idea what day that was, nor did I write it down. I think it was about day three. It remains such a blur.

I was hopeful yet annoyed each time the doctors would respond with, "We don't know," to my questions. I was happy that it wasn't a discouraging answer, yet I felt the need to want a tangible answer all at the same time.

We would get through one hurdle, only to have another hurdle rear its ugly head. I was given a blank book by a dear friend. As I read today what I wrote eight years ago, I am reminded how very fortunate we all really are, and that all the hurdles we actually jumped through successfully.

Mark was in Lee Memorial Hospital for fifteen days. We then transferred him to Sarasota to a rehab hospital where he spent the next thirty days. He woke up from his coma on March 11, 2010 which happened to be Fat Tuesday. New Orleans is our favorite city, so I found this to be fitting.

He then headed back to Lee Memorial for a cranioplasty to put the bone flap back in. I chartered a plane so that he could attend Shepherd Center in Atlanta. The Shepherd Center is a specialty hospital for spinal cord and brain injury. Mark ended up on the dual diagnostic ward because that was the only bed open at the time.

> "Mark eventually recovered from all of his injuries except his brain injury. That is something that we still manage on a daily basis."

Mark eventually recovered from all of his injuries except his brain injury. That is something that we still manage on a daily basis. Some days are good, and many are challenging. Hope is what keeps us going.

There were moments of setbacks and re-dos. I had to practice patience, patience and more patience. You get to know people and their stories while in these situations. You also come to know families of those who did not make it. Thank God we were the latter.

The moments turned into days, that turned into setbacks and high fives, joys, tears and at times downright discouragement. I did not have time to be sad, mad or angry. I had to be strong for Miracle Man Mark.

Sometimes I don't know how I managed through the last eight years. If we can do this, so can you!

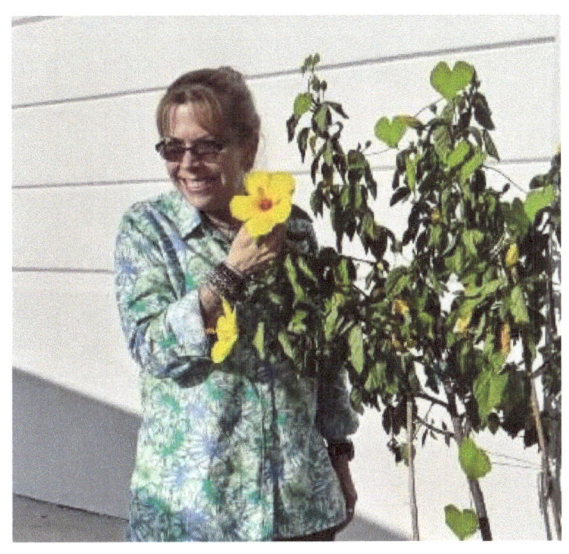

Meet Jackie Otto

Jackie Writes…

"My name is Jackie Otto, and I am a certified special education teacher of 25 years, and a lover of life. I had no idea how my training as a special educator would help me manage my life at home with a husband who has a Traumatic Brain Injury (TBI), and now we have a blind rescue dog named Slider, who acts as Mark's comfort dog."

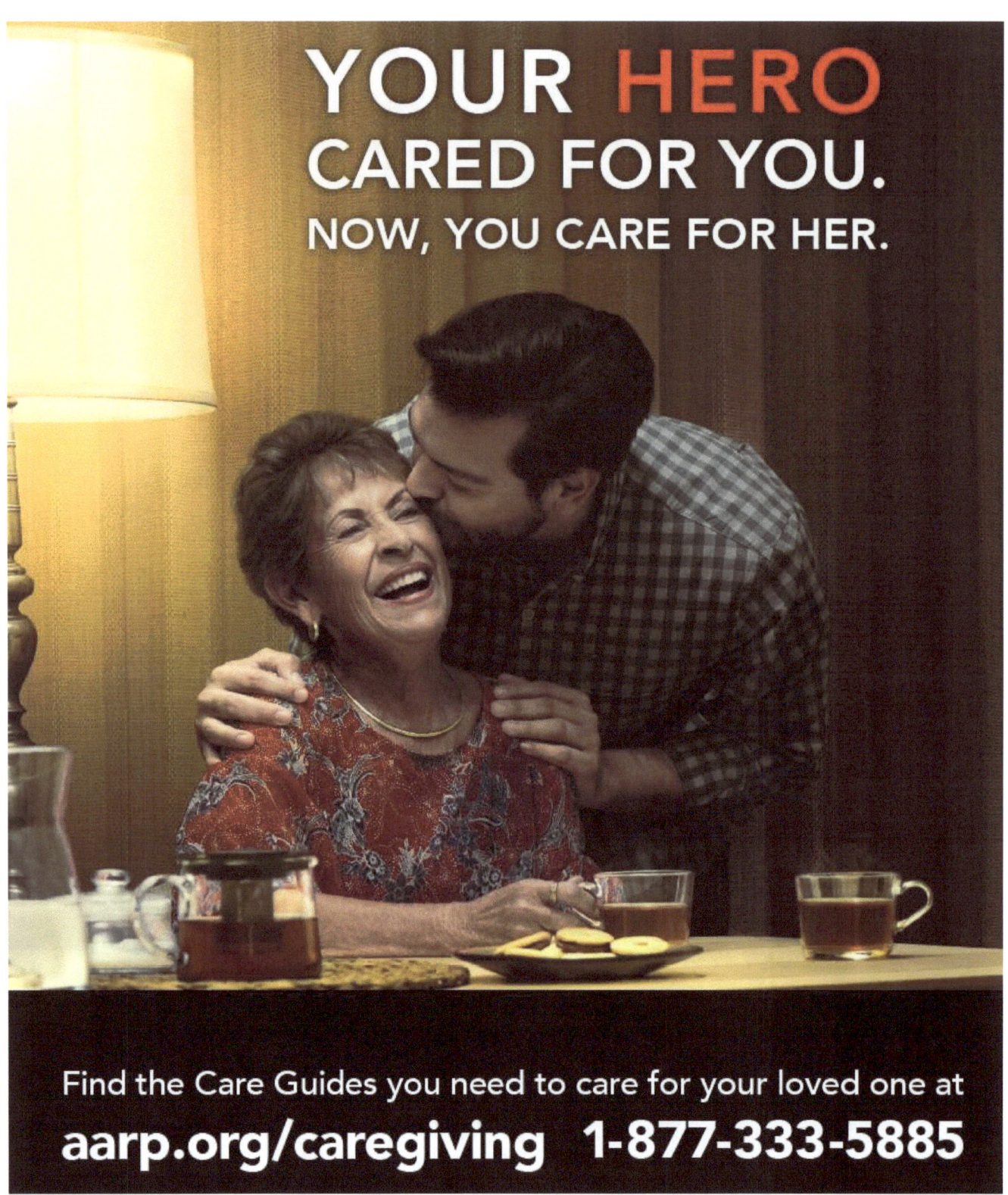

YOUR **HERO** CARED FOR YOU.

NOW, YOU CARE FOR HER.

Find the Care Guides you need to care for your loved one at

aarp.org/caregiving 1-877-333-5885

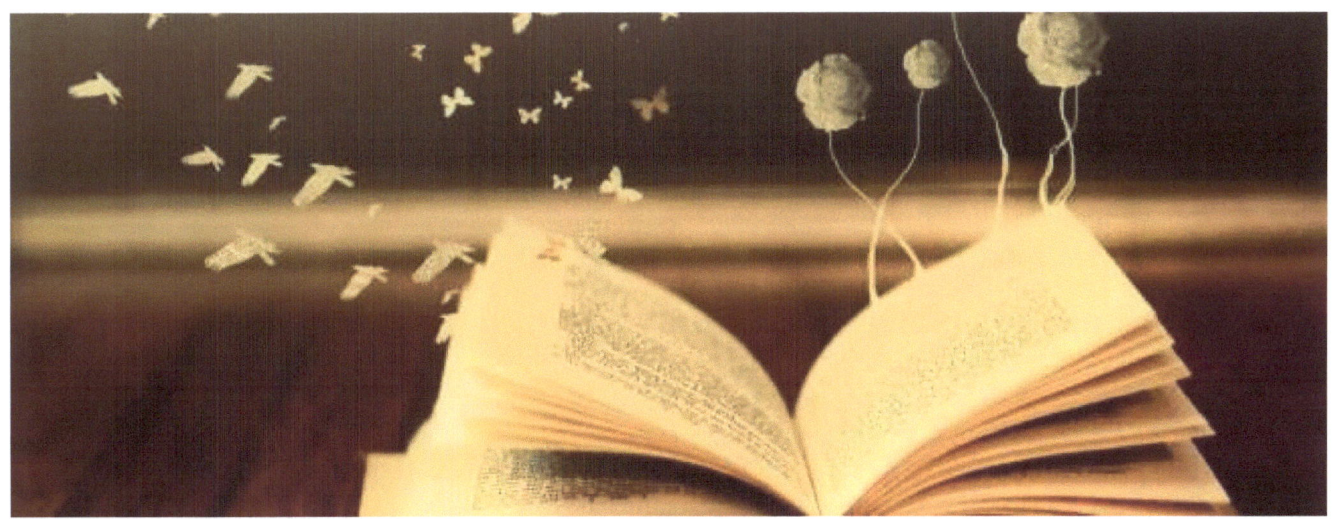

Saved by a Book

By Carmen Kumm

July 19, 2010 is my rebirthday. I was in a near fatal car accident with my two boys. We were headed to get my daughter at her friend's house. The driver that hit me says I never stopped, but I don't think I ever saw him. Others say it is a bad intersection and he was probably speeding and that's why I never saw him.

I call it my rebirthday because my life has changed completely. I was a high school Spanish teacher. After the accident, I was determined to get back to teaching if it was the last thing I did. I did return to teaching part-time in January.

> "After the accident, I was determined to get back to teaching if it was the last thing I did."

I finished that school year and thought I was back. To be honest, I cannot remember anything from that half of the year. By the fall I went back to teaching on a full-time basis.

My daughter was in my class at that time. She told me I was not as good a teacher as I had been before my accident, but as far as I knew I was back. The next year was about the same. On Monday of the first week in May of 2013, I knew by the beginning of that week that I was not going to make it through the end of week. Planning ahead, I took Friday off because of how I was feeling. During the last forty minutes of the day I had four sophomore boys being a pain and not working well with me.

I gave one of the boys a high five just like the V-8 commercials. He said that I had hit him, and he was going to go tell the principal. I told him to go ahead, knowing that I had done no wrong. Fifteen minutes later the day ended, and I went to the principal's office myself.

Much to my surprise, the principal suspended me for three days. We talked for a very long time. I was angry that he didn't know how far I had come. He was new that year, so he didn't know of my past successes as a teacher. I had been teaching for twenty-one years at that point and I had been an exemplary teacher. I had many students that went on to do many great things. It was during those three days that I took a good hard look at my life. I talked to my union representative as well as my family. I was able to see how badly my TBI was ruining my life. And quite bitterly, I decided to resign.

Shortly after my resignation, I took a trip to my local post office. Arriving five minutes before they opened, a help wanted sign caught my eye. It was for a position in a small town near where I live. It was only about twelve hours a week. I thought this was perfect, but the posting ended that day. When the postmaster came out, I asked her if she would consider hiring me if I applied. She said if I applied that she would indeed hire me as nobody else had applied. I went straight to the library to use the computer to apply. I was hired and trained in August.

For the next two years, I worked about twelve hours a week, then my job unexpectedly changed. In order to keep my job, I had to take a test. I've never practiced a test so much. It was a test on how you are able to figure things out and categorize things - not the easiest thing for a TBI person to do. But after three days of instruction, I passed the test without any problems. I was so excited!

> **"I was able to see how badly my TBI was ruining my life."**

I now work about twenty-five hours a week. I'm able to keep my house clean and enjoy my family. My girls are no longer living at home and my boys are in high school.

My youngest daughter was only ten years old at the time of my accident. She was very angry at me after the accident. We had our moments where I believed that she actually hated me. I will admit that I was not the nicest person to be around. Unfortunately, she received the brunt of my anger. We now get along much better and talk almost daily. She's in the USAF, stationed in Louisiana.

My sons were also young when the accident happened. For a long time, my youngest son was afraid of me and how I reacted to things. One of the first things I noticed the year after I quit teaching was his willingness him to come and sit with me and give me big hugs.

My husband has been wonderful. I really don't know how I would have done this without him. I know that he very easily could have left me and taken the kids, but he didn't. That's love.

These days, I still have short term memory issues. I need to write everything down or put it in my phone in order to remember it. There are also big chunks of my life that I just don't remember independently. Thank goodness for pictures. I also am very easily fatigued. I take a lot of naps and don't go out as much as I used to. I also don't do very well in large groups or in situations where things need to be done quickly.

I read a book named *Rebooting My Brain* by Maria Ross. It changed my life. What I took from that book changed how I looked at my accident and my life. My life wasn't over, it was just new. The old me had died and I needed to mourn her. The new me was reborn and just getting started. I know that I was meant to go to the post office that day and find that job. Better still, I know that the new me is going to be okay – no matter what.

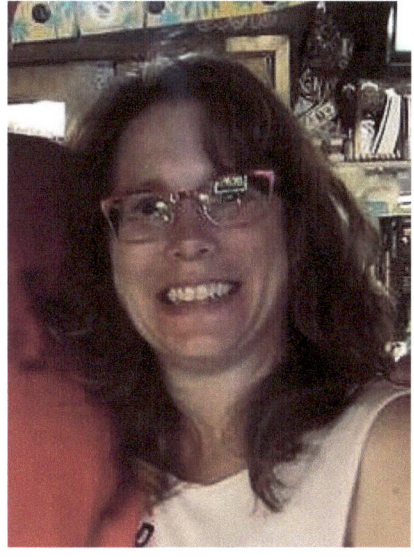

Meet Carmen Kumm

Originally from Bismarck, ND, Carmen received her bachelor's degree in secondary education. She moved to Pittsfield, WI in 1991 and married a couple of years later. She is the proud mom of four children and has done a remarkable job learning to live as a brain injury survivor since her 2010 traumatic brain injury.

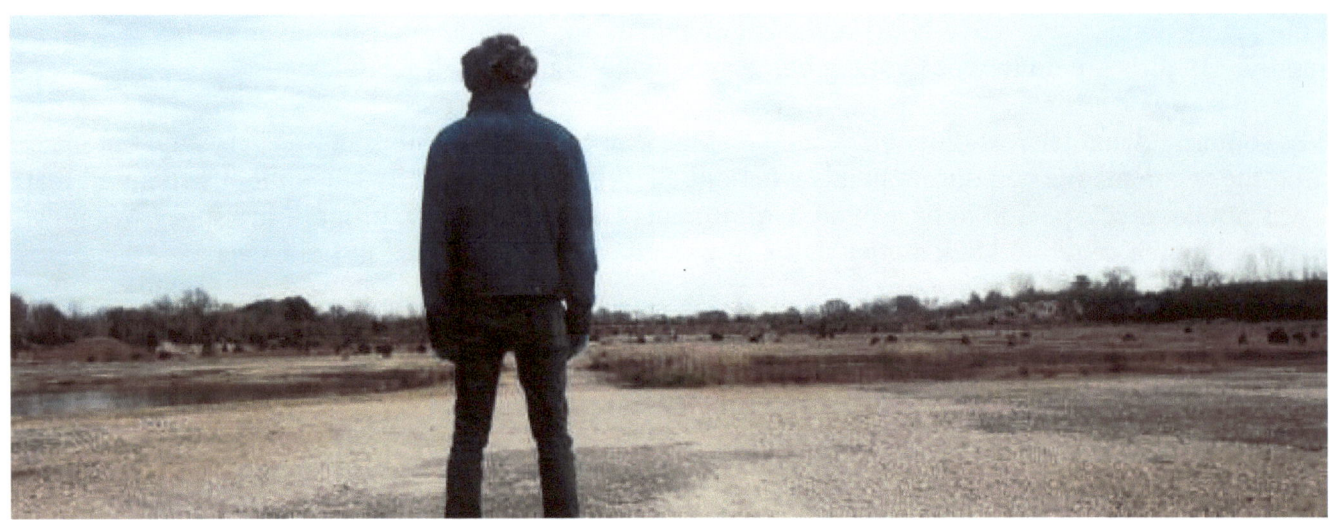

What Could Have Been

By Ventura Manzanares

My mother abandoned me on Christmas Eve in 1952, when I was only five weeks old. I was left at my stepdad's parent's house. I was raised by step-grandparents, and an alcoholic step-aunt.

My step-grandfather was alcoholic, had a stroke and died when I was six years old. I remember sitting by his bed in the back porch bedroom as he mumbled to me. My step-grandmother started abusing me when I was only four years old.

I was made to shovel coal into a broken cement furnace for five winters in Colorado. The dirt sunk under the weight of the twenty-five-year-old, handmade, concrete furnace. The flue had pulled

> "I was poisoned by long term, low level Carbon Monoxide gas from the age of four to nine years old."

away from the chimney. I was poisoned by long-term, low-level Carbon Monoxide gas from the age of four to nine years old. I ended up with an ABI (Acquired Brain Injury), that was undiagnosed and untreated for forty-nine years. I had an overwhelmed, hyper-vigilant brain.

Everything came in way too fast for me to process and cope with. I was unconscious about what was going on around me, like a fog, freeze frame or time delay. It was followed by C-PTSD, Complex or childhood post-traumatic stress disorder, from the abuse and the many deaths and losses in my life that followed.

I started getting cluster headaches when I was fifteen years old. They travelled from the back of my head to my eye, top to temple. I didn't know they were a side-effect of the carbon monoxide poisoning. I didn't even know that I had been poisoned, only that I never felt right in my mind. It was like a heavy weight on my head, face, and chest, like a dark cloud hanging on me. Some days I felt good, most days were in darkness and detachment. I have very little memory of my childhood or the first thirty years of my life. Christmas, birthdays, life in general, I have no real memory of.

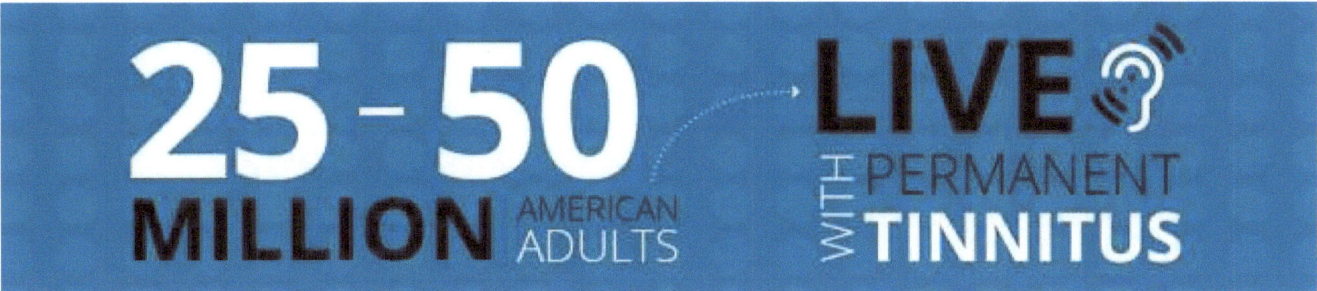

Another side-effect from the carbon monoxide poisoning is severe tinnitus. My ears ring all the time and have for as long as I can remember. It is the first thing I hear in the morning and the last thing at night, it's a constant throbbing, ringing in both ears, and it makes me crazy sometimes.

The mothers I had growing up through the school years were always someone else's mother. The neighbor, my friends' moms, some of my friends had two moms. I went through seven different families. No woman ever came into my life to be a real mother to me.

The neighbor girls up the street I was in high school with invited me to dinner one night, and their mother worked at Frontier Airlines. We talked about family. For fourteen years she worked with my

mother there, side by side, and she said to me, "She's never mentioned you." I meant nothing to my mother. She would not even speak my name.

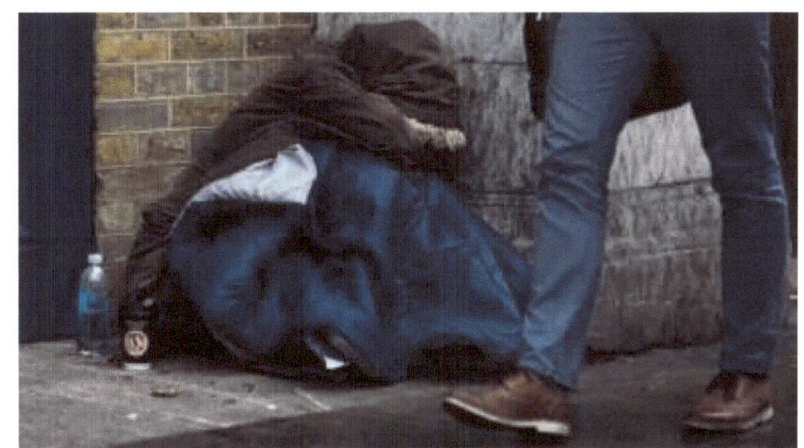

My brain was spinning out of control. I didn't know I was poisoning myself, owning a pest control company. I was compromising an already overwhelmed, hyper-vigilant, carbon monoxide brain. I couldn't deal with the stress or pressures of life. I felt pulled apart by the all of it.

I was homeless for five years in California. I found Safe Harbor shelter, in South San Francisco, in 2009 and got MediCal healthcare. I was properly diagnosed in 2011 for the carbon monoxide poisoning after forty-nine long years, by a psychiatrist doctor from India, who knew just what to do for me.

I was put on drug therapy for a full year until my white blood cell count crashed. He then took me off the treatment. It worked within days, changing the pathways in my brain and cleared my thought processes. It was like the first breath of fresh air for my brain. The spinning stopped, the dark heavy cloud lifted, and I got a lot smarter. I went through vocational rehabilitation and scored a 163 on the IQ test. I also went to mental health therapy, took the EMDR course for the C-PTSD, and I feel better to this day, and a lot happier.

It's living with the fallout from fifty years of detachment, spinning out of consciousness, plus blackout rage and anger, that linger on. I am not a survivor, I'm a warrior. Most people wouldn't last a day in my shoes or an hour in my head.

> **"I am not a survivor, I'm a warrior. Most people wouldn't last a day in my shoes or an hour in my head."**

I wake up every day, an orphaned, abandoned, unadopted, thrown away soul, and always feel alone, never knowing a mother's love, or comfort, or safety, but always feeling the abandonment and loss and knowing of all these mother's losses and their pains as well.

I live every day with mental illness and brain damage. I loved those close to me the best I knew how, and I cried for the rest. I am grateful for the love I've received and the pain I carry. I am truly sorry my heart, soul and brain were so badly damaged.

Sometimes I find myself wondering what could have been…

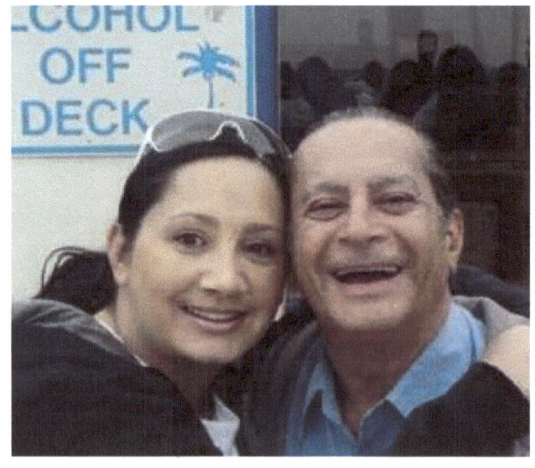

Meet Ventura Manzanares

Ventura is a self-described TBI Warrior. Over the years he has found that attitude is indeed everything as he strives to move through his life with grace, dignity and honor. He continues to work hard on his recovery and hopes that his story will inspires others to know that they to can overcome what seem like insurmountable odds.

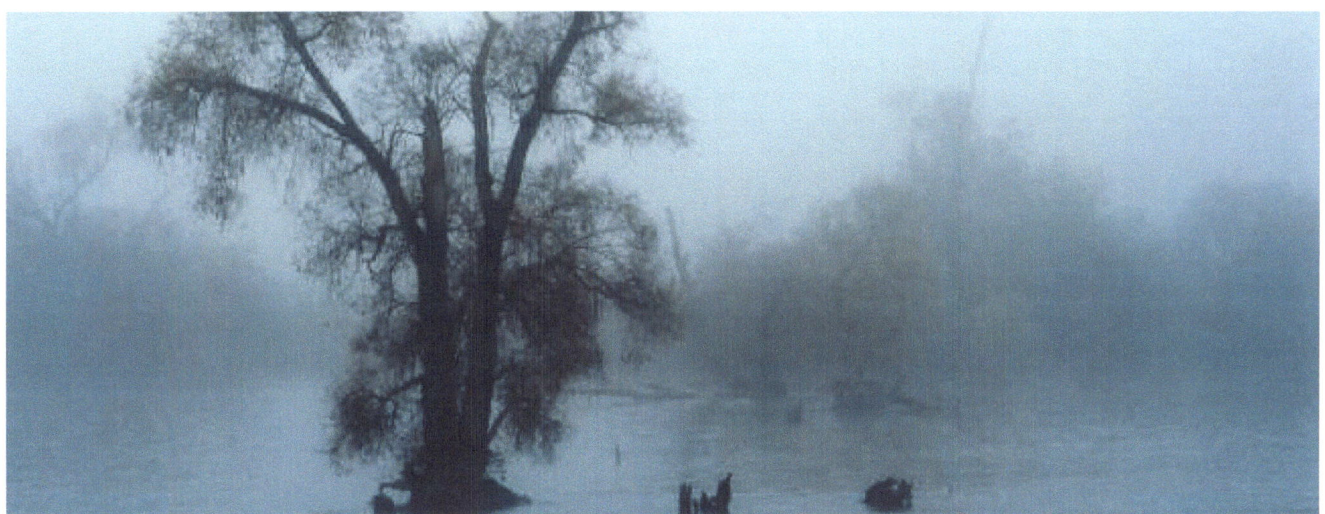

Out of the Smoke

By Cole Taylor

I've been living with a traumatic brain injury for five years. I am now beginning to look ahead. What I look forward to must be better than what I have experienced. I've spent five years dealing with lost executive function, corrupted visual processing, PTSD, physical injuries and with chronic pain. I had an inability to manage day-to-day affairs, and experienced job losses, and more.

Seemingly overnight, people I loved, cared for and supported simply abandoned me. Perhaps they thought that I was so self-sufficient that they couldn't imagine my needing help. Perhaps they were frightened that the same thing would happen to them if they associated with me.

> "How I've survived all of this, why I did not die of my injuries or confusion or loneliness or fear I'll never know."

I've been abused and lied to and about by people I trusted. My life isn't helped by society's perception that an overweight older widow is worthless. But brain injured too? It's like having an invisibility cloak. How I've survived all of this, why I did not die of my injuries, or confusion, or loneliness, or fear I'll never know.

How I did not accidentally overdose because I couldn't read the pill bottles or commit suicide out of despair, remains a mystery. This is a mystery that leads to questions: How do I construct a life that will allow me to thrive? How do I lead a life that fulfills the purpose I've yet to find?

Inventorying what skills I have left, relative to those I used to have, is not helpful. Nothing depresses me more than looking back at what might have been, unless it's surveying the smoking ruins of my future.

It's time for a mountain-top view, to get out of the smoke, and to look towards a new and fresh horizon. I'm going to take out a pen and paper and start a new list. Maybe, a new life. It's now time to focus on the Zen of this new life. All I have is this moment, a moment I need to fully experience. It's my time to find joy where possible. I will wait for the pain to pass when necessary.

I can learn to trust, yet still protect. I can learn to wait and to watch. Motives and intentions are not always what they seem. Knowing this brings freedom.

Respect others' thoughts and behaviors as being entirely their own. They are not a reflection on my worth or worthiness. Forgive, set aside the hurt, move forward. Step-by-step I will shed resentments while finding my new path.

By becoming an intrepid inventor, I will find ways of doing what will work for me now. I will develop ways of being and of creating that will support continued healing and bring about a peaceful spirit.

I will choose to remember compassion and practice consideration, while not sacrificing my well-being to do it.

Be still and know there is a God, who works all things for the good of those who love Him.

The smoke will clear, I'll see the path, and know this is true.

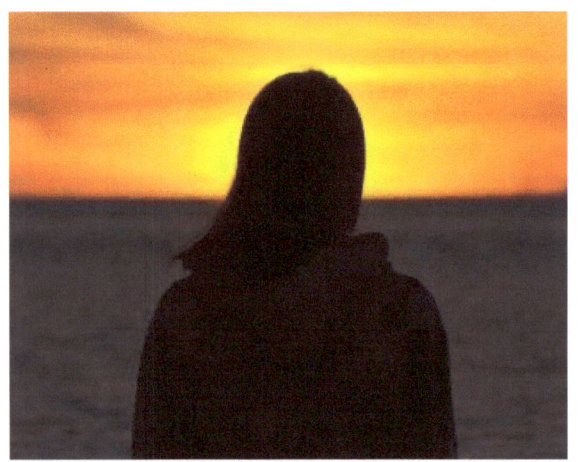

About Cole Taylor

In 2014, Cole tripped and fell, hitting her head on a counter and again on the floor. She suffered coup-contrecoup, diffuse axonal and visual cortex damage, along with jaw, neck, and back injuries. Our contributor has asked that we publish her story under her pen name of Cole Taylor citing safety concerns of living in a small town as a brain injury survivor.

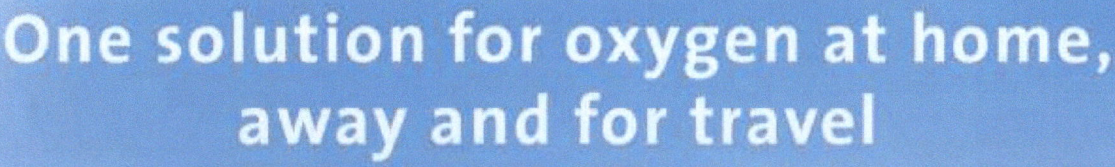
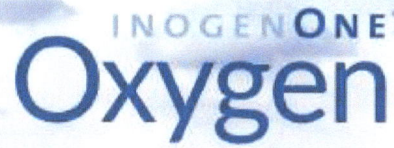

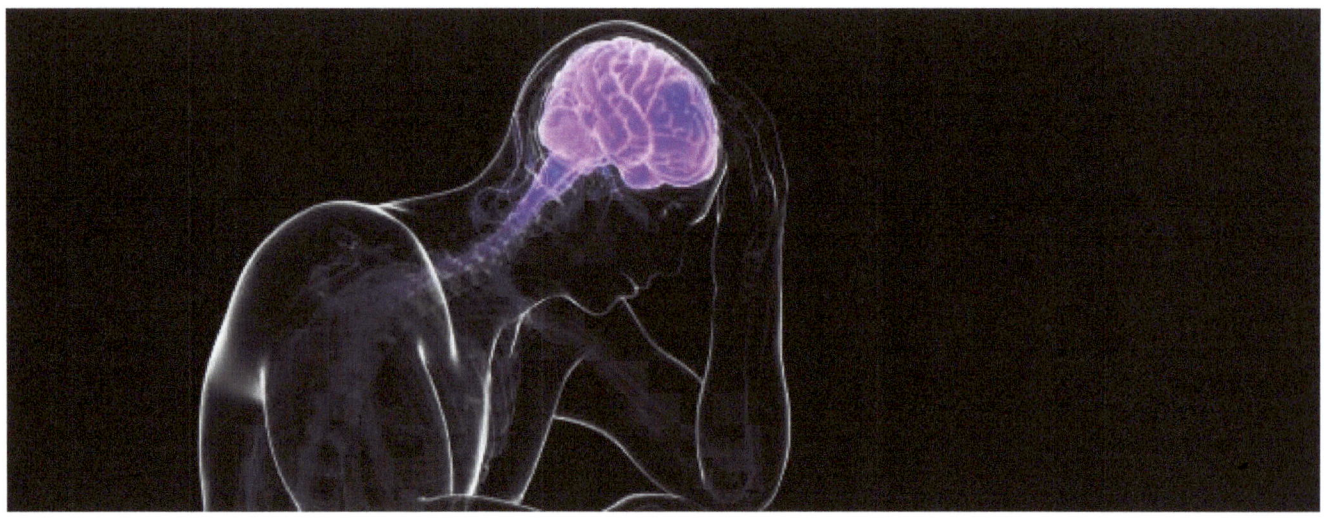

Brain Injury and Mental Illness

By Christopher Jay

For almost thirty years I unknowingly labored under the effects of traumatic brain injuries; documented, undocumented, and some, only uncovered decades later after suffering yet another traumatic brain injury. Even after waking from a brief coma and being given CT scan images of pre-existing brain damage, my wife and I remained ill-informed about my injuries, uneducated about the severity and recovery, and left unknowingly to travel along the very same, progressively worsening path that would have me twice involuntarily hospitalized several years after my fourth TBI.

Each of my brain injuries is considered medically mild to moderate, but the consequences have been anything but moderate, exacerbated by each additional trauma. To this extent, my recovery did not begin until I found several thousand individuals with similar injuries from all walks of life, including medical doctors, located within private Facebook Groups.

> "Each of my brain injuries is considered medically mild to moderate, but the consequences have been anything but moderate, exacerbated by each additional trauma."

Only then, through reading, responding, posting, and sharing experiences and symptoms with survivors of trauma, stroke, tumor, drowning, etcetera, did I truly start to understand that the injuries manifested in my head were anything but invisible or character flaws.

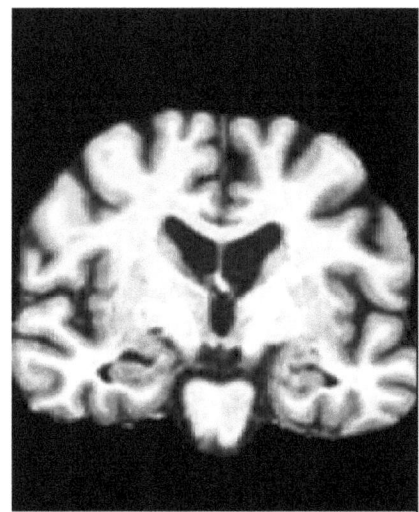

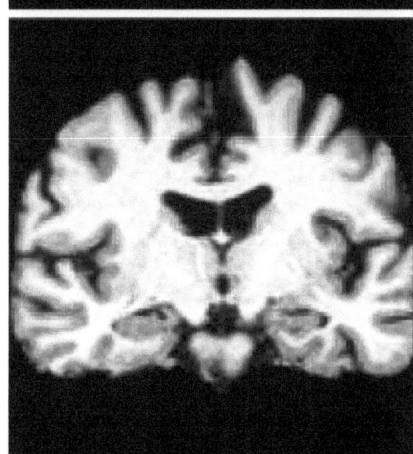

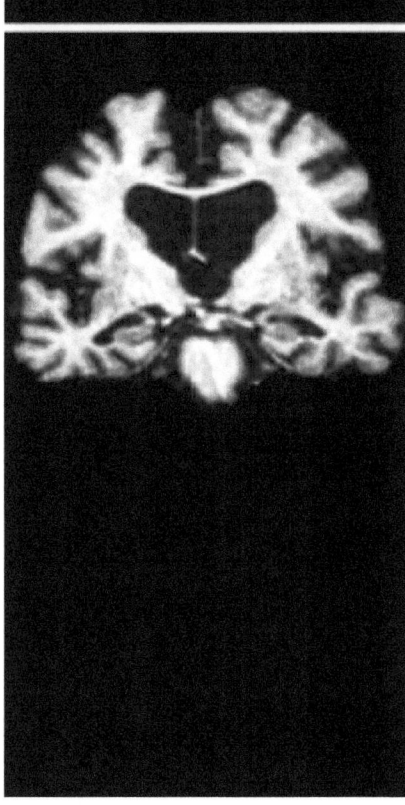

Brain injuries can cause mental illnesses, most commonly severe depression. However, under no circumstances is that fate a forgone conclusion, nor is there a conclusive list of mental illnesses that brain injuries can cause.

It is imperative to understand that the majority of the approximately 1.4 million Americans that annually experience a traumatic brain injury, will recover and resume their normal lives. Nonetheless, approximately 20% or 275,000 of those annually injured will find themselves at a foggy intersection, with or without mental illness.

For these millions of individuals amassed over the years, the symptoms are bewildering, destructive to their own lives as well as marriages and family, and provide a never-ending patient pool that is poorly understood and often misdiagnosed by the medical and psychological professions.

It is critical that we as parents, survivors and caregivers understand that brain injuries impact millions more than our professional football players, whose stories now grace the silver screen. More newsworthy, traumatic brain injuries are not restricted to a singular sport or level of achievement. Rather, they are an integral part of being human and can be caused by falling off a roof, motor vehicle accidents, domestic violence, playing soccer, slipping on ice, cheerleading, drunk driving, riding a bicycle, skiing, etc.

Moreover, brain injuries are not restricted to the 1.4 million who annually suffer *trauma.* Every year within our borders, an additional one million individuals suffer an *acquired* brain injury (ABI), causing many of the same symptoms. These result from brain tumors, strokes, drownings, aneurysms, smoke inhalation, meningitis, seizure disorder, and so forth.

Our children, our families, and each of us need to understand that brain injuries do not occur in vacuums nor are they mutually exclusive from all of life's other injuries and ailments, including mental illness. Thus, it may be impossible to clear the fog from the intersection, leaving many unable to determine if mental illness preceded a brain injury or if brain injury brought about a mental illness, such as Bi-Polar Disorder.

Survivors of any brain injury, along with their doctors, are, thus, often left treating a myriad of symptoms most of which exist silently within a person's brain, yet govern all of their emotions, pain, behavior, judgment – all that encompasses the human experience. However, we can do much better by encouraging collaboration, communication and the exchange of information between the numerous medical sub-specialties and various psychological camps. Furthermore, I implore the medical profession to provide better written information about what a brain injury encompasses, including how to best maximize short and long term recovery and what future warning signs a survivor, and especially their family, should be aware of.

Lastly, an injured brain may result in a diseased brain. However, I refuse to accept that my injured brain cannot be successfully treated. Even when utterly hopeless and consumed by desperation, hope remains, if only we commit to steadfastly searching. In addition to the kindness and compassion of my family and friends, much of the hope that I desperately cling to came from complete strangers living with brain injuries and/or mental illness, most of whom I met online. My life is enriched as a direct result of these unexpected friendships, and for that, I will be forever grateful.

Meet Christopher Jay

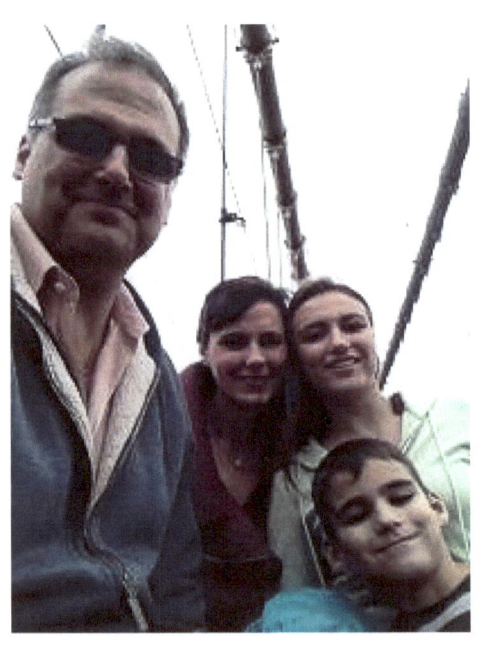

Christopher has survived six brain injuries spread across his 52 years, the last being eleven years ago, resulting in a brief coma. He lives in New York with his wife, daughter and son. He credits the support of his small family nucleus as the largest part of his motivation to continue his recovery.

Christopher is equally grateful to his Facebook friends and acquaintances, with whom he credits helping him find his unique understanding and answers for his injuries, as all who are injured and ill are unique. In celebrating his recovery, Chris and his family are finally launching their new business, BlanketPals.com. Chris wishes all survivors, care-givers, and loved one's peace, kindness and genuine gratitude.

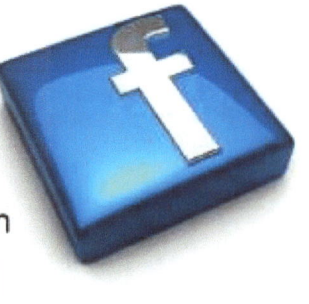

A Ghost Among Mortals

By Bode McKay

Life on hold
How do I even explain?
How can you understand
What goes through my head
Each and every day?
A thousand lies
Torment my mind
Make me feel beaten,
Broken, alone,
Dread, fear,
Scream, weary.
I fight a war
Long after my war ended.
A war of the mind
Battle for control
Struggle to let go.
Visions so real
They bring me to my knees.
Peeking around every corner
For the threat I cannot see.
Having a plan to hurt someone
If they try to hurt me.
Hating people more and more
Eyes roll at their petty problems.
Contemplating the abyss
The vast emptiness
Full of hopelessness.
It has a name
And no one knows
Unless you have it.
It sounds harmless
But nonetheless
It is dangerous
To the mind and soul.
TBI
No one understands.
I am a ghost among mortals
Invisible because they cannot see
The monster inside me.
I want to connect, to love, to move on,
But it slaps me back into my place
And there I am
On the floor
Back at square one.
TBI
What it means to you
Is not the same to me.
You see fine
I feel pain.

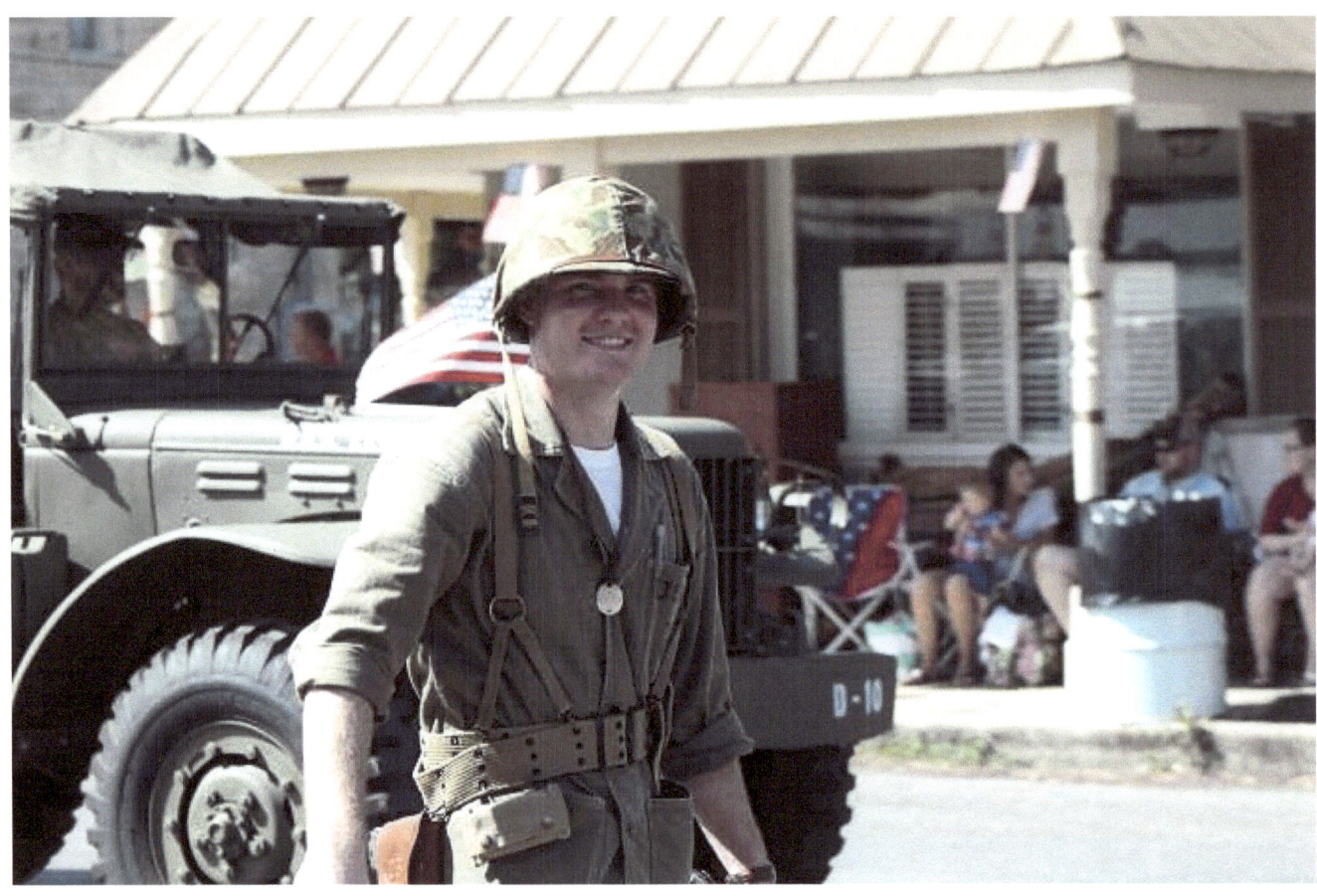

Bode's Story

By Debbie McKay

Editor's Note: When we received the poem that you've just read from Bode's mom Debbie, we reached out to her asking for a bio to accompany his powerful poem. Debbie sent over Bode's story. His story was so compelling that we opted to share the details of his story with you.

Bode McKay knew what he wanted to do since he was five years old when he played Abe Lincoln in his kindergarten play. From that moment on a spark was ignited and he spent the rest of his young life reading, studying and learning anything and everything he could about history.

As a young boy, Bode befriended a World War II veteran named Ben Parish and the two became great friends. He shared his experiences with Bode. This was when Bode realized that he wanted to dedicate his life to honor our veterans and the sacrifices they made so that future generations would never forget.

He was so focused on his goals that he decided to fast track his education and was able to finish high school by age sixteen. He went on to get his BA by the age of eighteen and was in grad school at age nineteen, at the time of his incident.

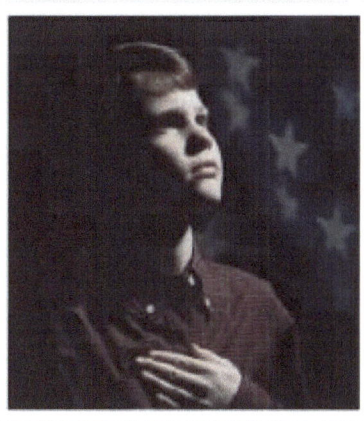 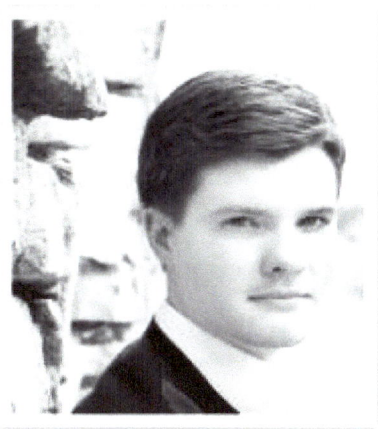 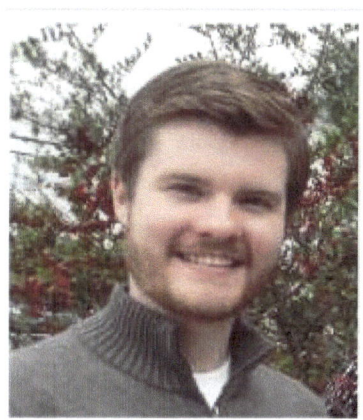

As a young boy, Bode visited a local World War II museum and dreamed of one day being involved with their living history program. When he turned fifteen that is exactly what he did and was also able to spend several years traveling the state and bringing history to life.

On August 30, 2014 his young life changed forever. During one of the reenactments at the museum, two men made the decision to drag and place Bode over a pyrotechnic charge that subsequently exploded on his head. As a result, Bode received a Traumatic Brain Injury, PTSD, multiple other injuries and disorders.

Life as he knew it stopped from that day forward and has been spent searching for the right medical care and trying to find a new purpose in his life. The old Bode's passion was history, but the new Bode wanted nothing to do with it anymore and developed new creative outlets that were nonexistent before.

Among these are writing, drawing, art and poetry. Using a computer is difficult for him as there are so many distractions, so his parents bought him an old typewriter and that is where he finds himself most happy when he is sitting in front of it typing out poetry and stories.

The road has been long and difficult and there is still a long way to go, but Bode continues to see improvements each and every day as he merges the old and new Bode together and hopes to one day be able to go back to school, become a history professor, and continue his life's mission.

Although the world is full of suffering, it is also full of the overcoming of it.

~Helen Keller

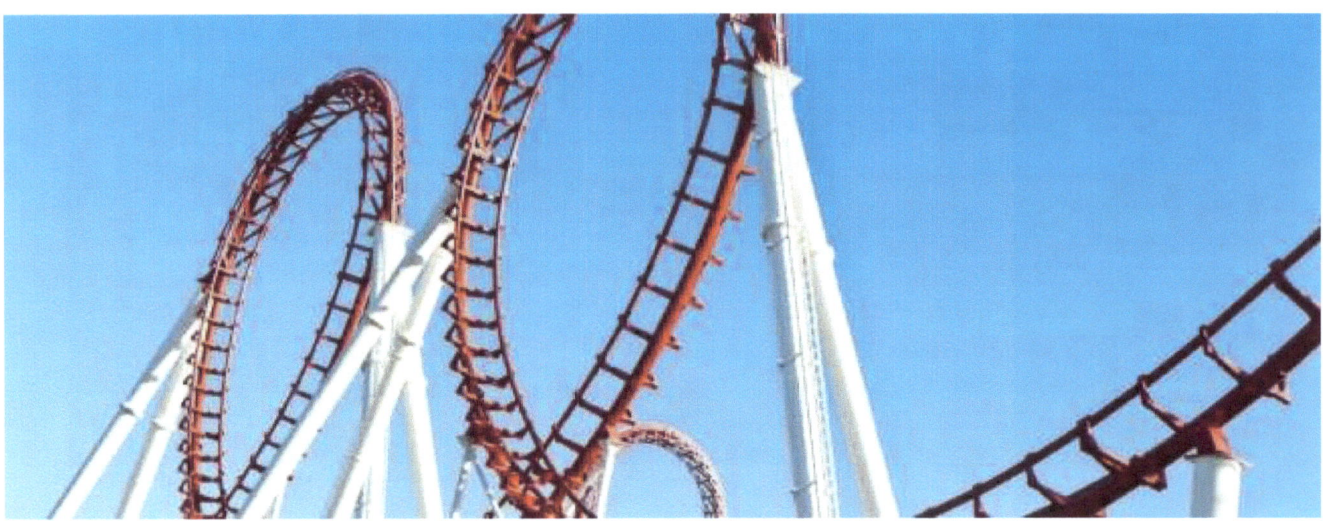

The Brain Injury Roller Coaster
By Ted Stachulski

As the summer heats up, my family members get more excited about going away on a week-long vacation with another family to Hampton Beach on the seacoast of New Hampshire. While they are all planning the things they want to do on vacation, I plan ways that I can reserve my energy and scope out places where I can take twenty-minute naps to recharge my batteries.

When I've gone away on vacation with just my family members, my fatigue only affected them and their plans. However, since this upcoming vacation is with another family, I worry about what they want to do and how my fatigue is going to affect them.

I might have to explain to everyone that living with a brain injury is like being on a roller coaster. One day is an "up day" for me where I have energy in the morning to keep up with everyone, but I will need to take my nap in the afternoon so then I can keep up with everyone in the evening. I'll then have to explain to them that the following day will be a "down day" and I'll need to rest all day to recharge my batteries.

> "When I've gone away on vacation with just my family members, my fatigue only affected them and their plans."

On the "down days" I feel more mentally tired with brain fog, dizzy, and not my happy self. I'm moodier and get bothered by things that really shouldn't bother me. I have more double vision and walk into things like the corner of a table or a doorway. I drop more things out of my left hand and can trip while walking more easily. I definitely need to take more frequent naps and need to avoid any risky or dangerous activities for my own safety.

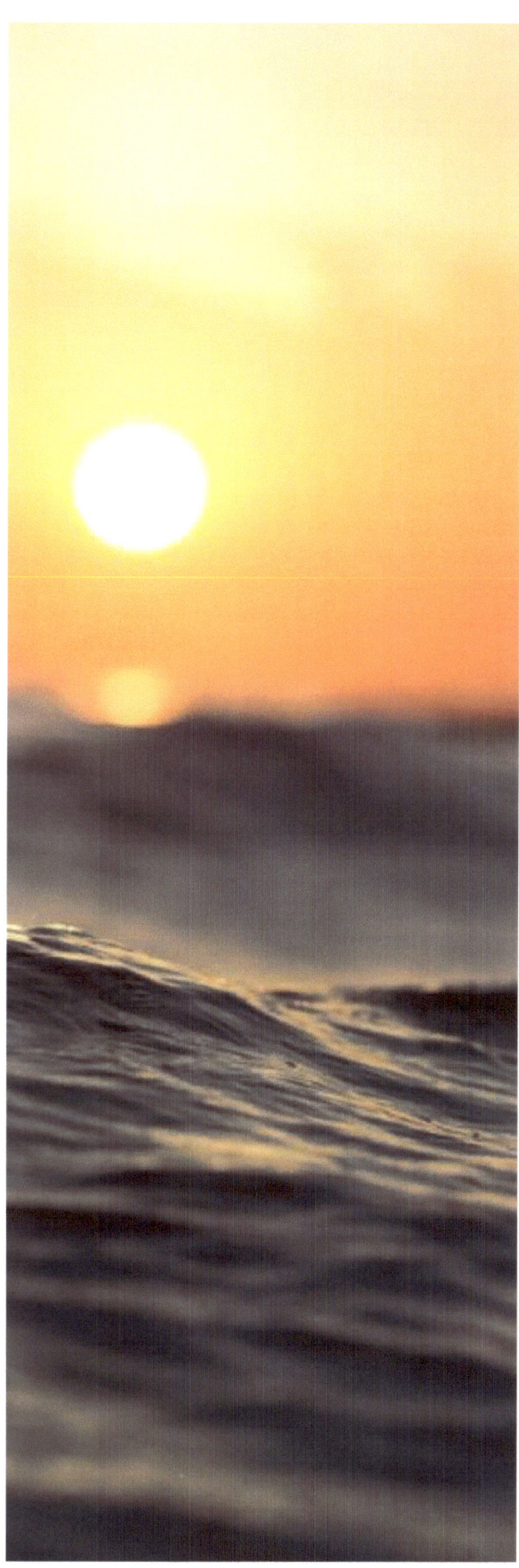

Sometimes my family members are okay with me needing to take more breaks and naps, while sometimes it bothers them. Sometimes they are okay with me staying at the cottage by myself while they go off and explore and enjoy the scenery and activities, and at other times, they are not.

Sometimes I push myself two days in a row without taking a day off, but that means the next two days will be "down days." When I get home from vacation, I'll need at least a week to recover, even though I was on vacation. The bottom line is that I pay a price for playing.

Keep in mind that living this way doesn't mean your vacation will be a horrible experience. My family members and I have had fun over the years visiting places like Old Orchard Beach and Boothbay Harbor in Maine. We've been to Lake Winnipesaukee and Clark's Trading Post in New Hampshire, visited the USS Constitution and walked the Freedom Trail in Massachusetts. The key is planning ahead as much as possible and accepting that you will need to take a break after deciding to do something spontaneously.

My down time is time for me and my family members to reflect on how far I've come in my recovery. I couldn't go on vacation or even look at amusement park rides for over a decade after my brain injury because I got so overloaded by the sights, sounds, and other things. I've come a long way.

This is a testament to my family and I persevering and never giving up when things got tough. It's a tribute to all of my doctors, therapists, and friends I've made at brain injury support groups who helped me and my family members along our journey of recovery.

I still can't drink a beer with friends at a bar or go on some amusement park rides with them, but I can enjoy our friendship and take pictures of us having fun while both of our families create and share wonderful times together that will forever be engrained in our memories.

At times, it's hard for even the most seasoned family members and caregivers of brain injury survivors to understand this roller coaster concept.

So, whether you are going on vacation or planning a series of rehabilitation appointments this summer, keep in mind you or a loved one with a brain injury need to rest and recharge their batteries after a day of fun in the sun or at a rehabilitation facility. Doing so will make living this brain injured life on a roller coaster a little more tolerable and a lot more fun.

Have a fun and safe summer!

Meet Ted Stachulski

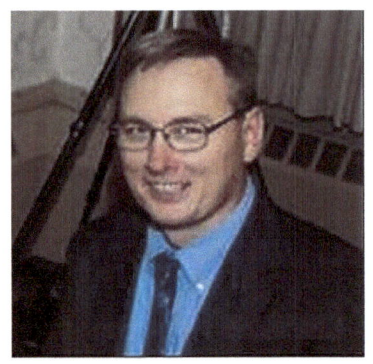

Ted Stachulski is a former multi-sport athlete, Marine Corps Veteran, Traumatic Brain Injury Survivor, and creator of the Veterans Traumatic Brain Injury Survivor Guide. Ted is also a Veterans Outreach Specialist and an advocate for brain injury survivors, their family members and caregivers. You can learn more about Ted at www.TBITed.com

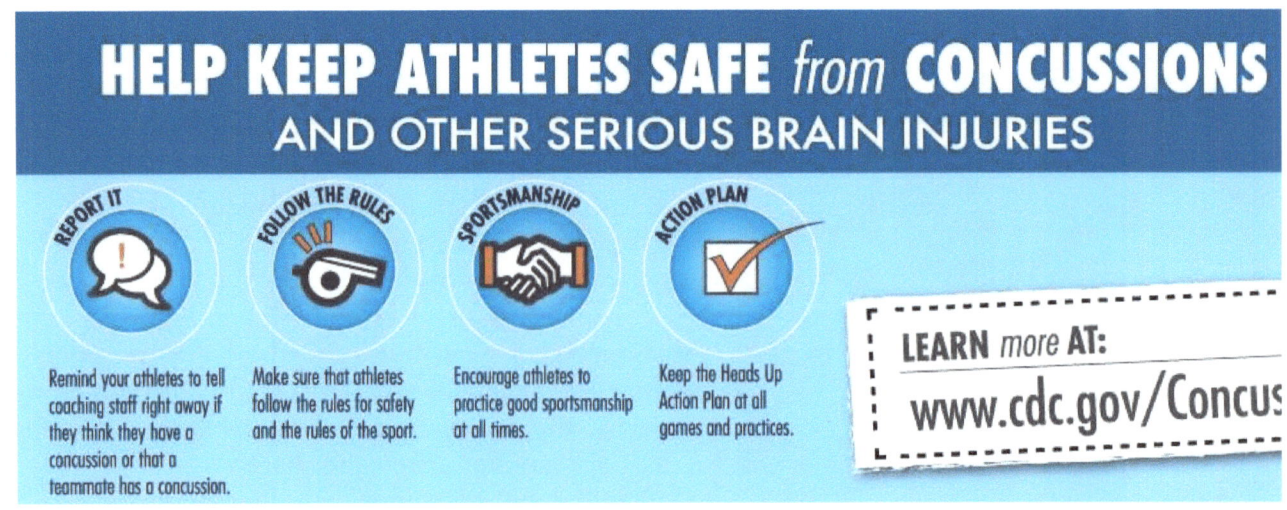

HELP KEEP ATHLETES SAFE *from* **CONCUSSIONS**
AND OTHER SERIOUS BRAIN INJURIES

REPORT IT — Remind your athletes to tell coaching staff right away if they think they have a concussion or that a teammate has a concussion.

FOLLOW THE RULES — Make sure that athletes follow the rules for safety and the rules of the sport.

SPORTSMANSHIP — Encourage athletes to practice good sportsmanship at all times.

ACTION PLAN — Keep the Heads Up Action Plan at all games and practices.

LEARN *more* AT:
www.cdc.gov/Concus

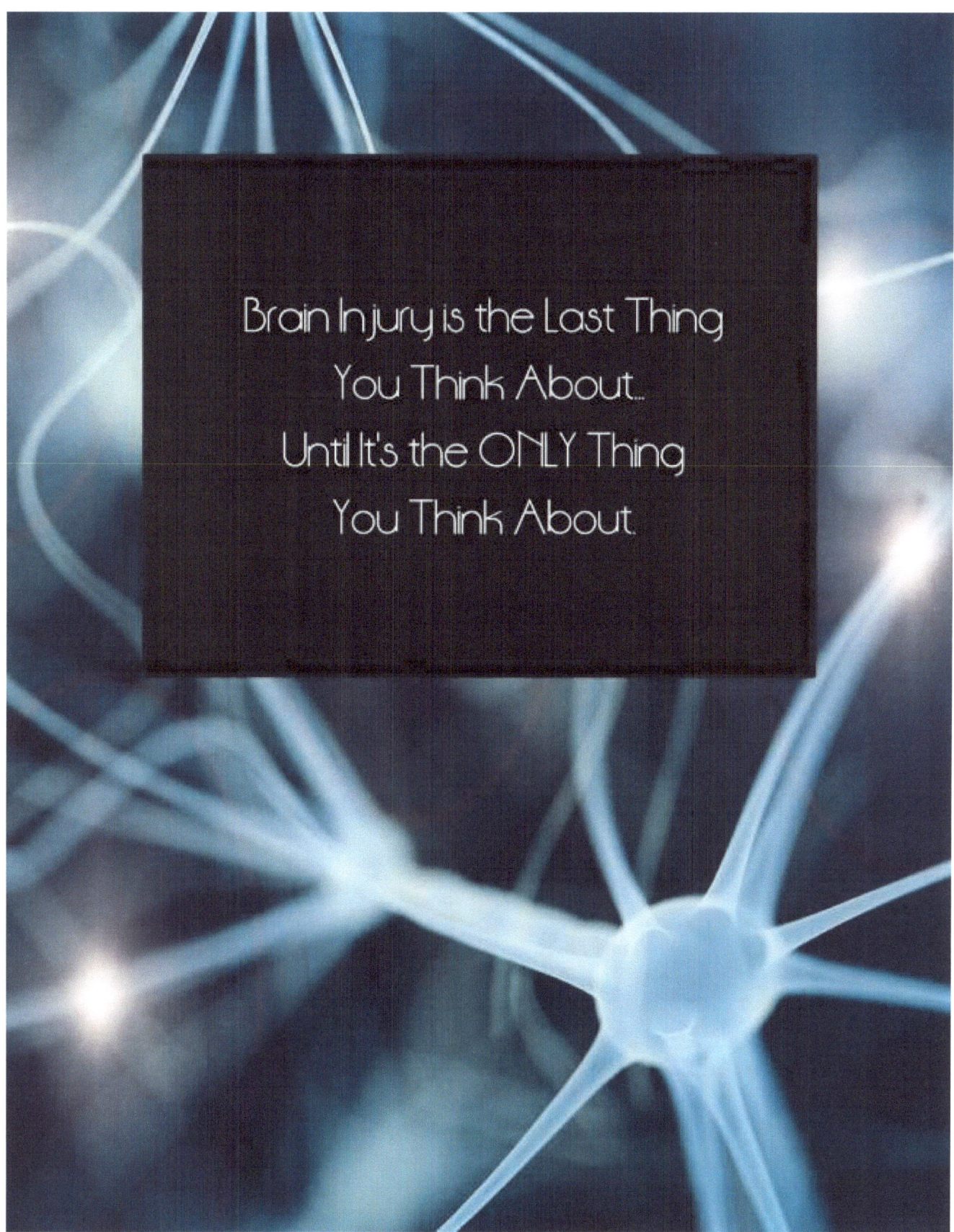

Brain Injury is the Last Thing
You Think About...
Until It's the ONLY Thing
You Think About.

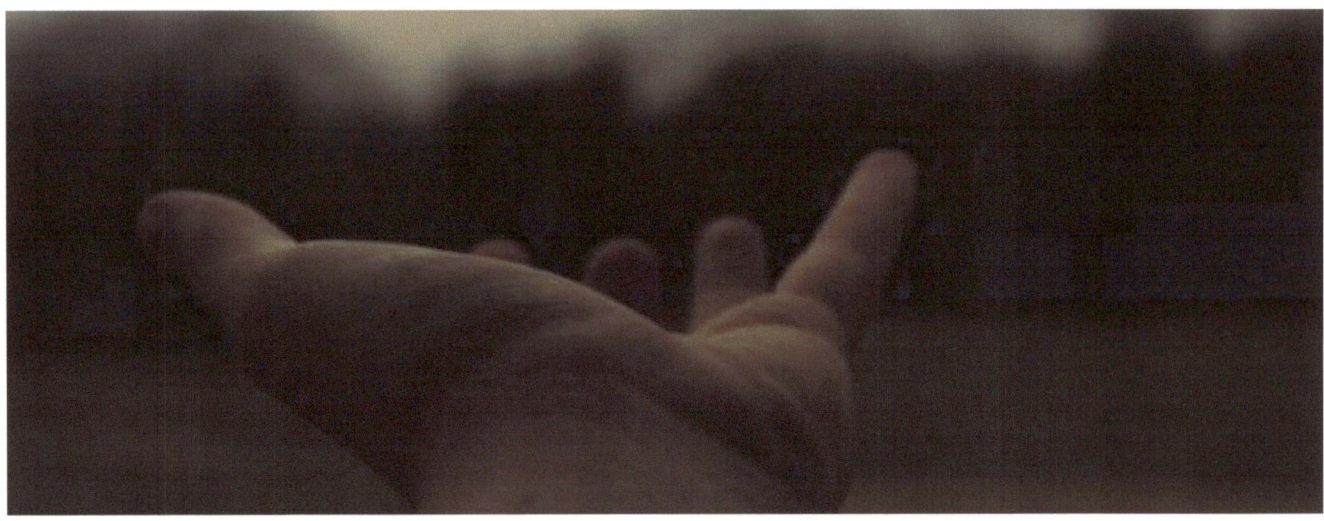

Becoming a Support Group Person

By Barbara Webster

I never thought I was a "support group person." I thought support groups were more for people who wanted to talk about their problems instead of doing something about them. In 1991, when a car skidded into mine on a slippery road and my life was turned upside down, little did I know that a support group would be one of the best things that ever happened to me. I looked okay after the accident, no obvious head wound, but inside I was far from okay.

Prior to my accident, I was a problem-solving, multitasking, goal-oriented, career woman, wife and mother. Now I struggled with simple everyday tasks - and I didn't know why! It felt like I was going crazy. After over two years of confusion, frustration and despair, I attended a program at my son's school featuring a speaker from the Brain Injury Association of Massachusetts. I remember trying to hide the tears that ran down my cheeks as I listened and finally realized that I was not alone.

> "I remember trying to hide the tears that ran down my cheeks as I listened and finally realized that I was not alone!"

I have been participating in brain injury support groups ever since, first as a member and later as a facilitator. I still remember the person who greeted me at those first meetings. That simple, friendly gesture was the highlight of my week that was otherwise filled with frustration and failure as I tried and failed to do the things that I used to be able to do with such ease. Support groups also helped my husband understand that I wasn't "losing it," and that I had a problem. We began to work together. They literally saved my marriage.

What I continue to hear regularly from support group members is that the most important benefit of a support group is in finding a place where you feel comfortable, where people "get it" and truly understand your issues. No need to explain yourself, apologize or make excuses, you are accepted and understood as you are. What will probably surprise you is all of the additional ways that I found a brain injury support group to be helpful.

I discovered strategies through support group members, those amazing little tools that help you do something you couldn't do otherwise. I love strategies! Each one feels like a little light bulb inside my head, an "aha moment," a mini miracle! Instead of dwelling on all of the things that I couldn't do, I began thinking about how to do them. I began to feel hopeful.

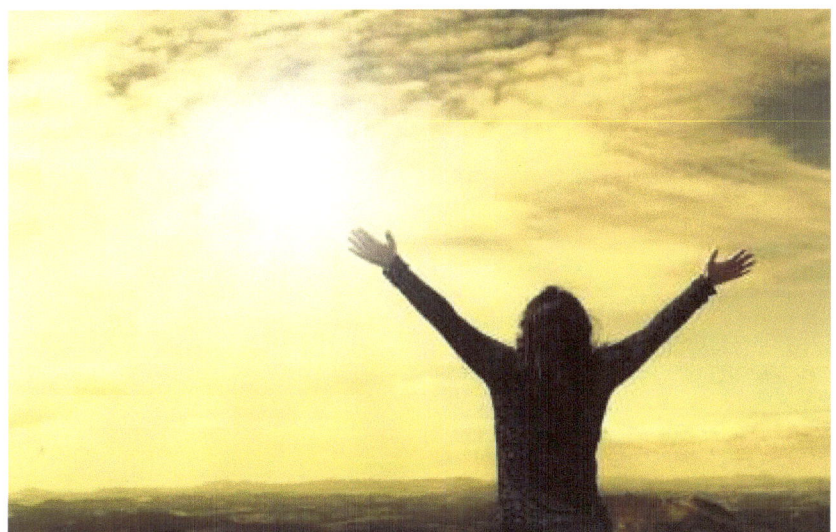

It was through support groups I discovered that there were professionals who could actually help me. I learned that there was such a thing as cognitive rehabilitation. What a revelation. What a relief. Those therapists, my "earth angels," helped me start the long process of putting my life back together. Finally, I had HOPE!

I think the most unexpected benefit of participating in a support group is the inspiration I received from observing other survivors accomplish things I wouldn't have considered doing before I witnessed their successes. Time and time again, I still find myself thinking: 'If they can do it, I should at least try, maybe I can do it too!' We inspire confidence and courage in each other just by witnessing each other's journeys.

Healing from a brain injury takes a long time. My insurance coverage and therapies stopped long before I was ready, and I would have been lost if I had not been part of a support group. My support group helped fill the gap. Most brain injury support groups offer much more than a forum for listening and sharing. They can also provide educational, recreational and social opportunities. They can be a place to make new friends. They can be a place to volunteer, providing a safe environment to practice skills and challenge your abilities. They are also a link to your state Brain Injury Associations, connecting you to resources statewide.

We were about to lose our facilitator and our support group when I took a leap of faith and volunteered to be the facilitator. I still don't know how I had the courage. In the beginning I just tried to give everyone an opportunity to share. Gradually, as I felt more capable, I composed monthly newsletters and invited an occasional guest speaker. Before long I was developing resource lists, arranging social and recreational activities and organizing projects. Running the group became my vehicle for rehabilitation. I could work on it at home, at my own pace, when the house was quiet, and I was having a "good brain day." The more I challenged myself, the more I redeveloped my skills and promoted my own rehabilitation process. Talk about unexpected benefits!

When I have a problem, I try to educate myself about it as much as possible. Well, there wasn't much information about brain injury available to educate myself with when I acquired my brain injury in 1991. We were starving for any information related to brain injury in the support group and eager to share anything that might be useful to us. Gradually more information became accessible. I began writing up my notes from our meetings, workshops & conferences I attended; organizing it for myself and for future meetings, adding to it as I learned more and more. Eventually, my collection of tips, tools, and strategies became a book to help other people with brain injury.

Brain injury survivors and their caregivers have a special wisdom, a wisdom gained from unique experiences, priceless to others in similar situations. My book is intended to help share this special wisdom with others who are living with brain injury and make their journey just a little bit easier.

Support groups aren't for everyone, but everyone needs support after something as traumatic and life changing as a brain injury. To find a support group in your area, please contact your state Brain Injury Association. It could be one of the best things that ever happens to you!

Meet Barbara Webster

Barbara Webster is the long-time facilitator of the Amazing Brain Injury Survivor Support Group in Framingham, MA and the Survivor and Family Educator for the Brain Injury Association of Massachusetts. Originally a teacher, Barbara's brain injury brought her back to her passion of being an educator and a mentor. It became her mission to encourage survivors to continue their healing and rehabilitation process, to inspire hope. Barbara is the author of a strategy workbook for survivors: Lost and Found, A Survivor's Guide for Reconstructing Life After a Brain Injury, as well as a contributing author to Chicken Soup for the Soul: Recovering from Traumatic Brain Injuries. Many of her articles are featured on www.brainline.org and some of her materials are being used by The Wounded Warrior Project supporting veterans.

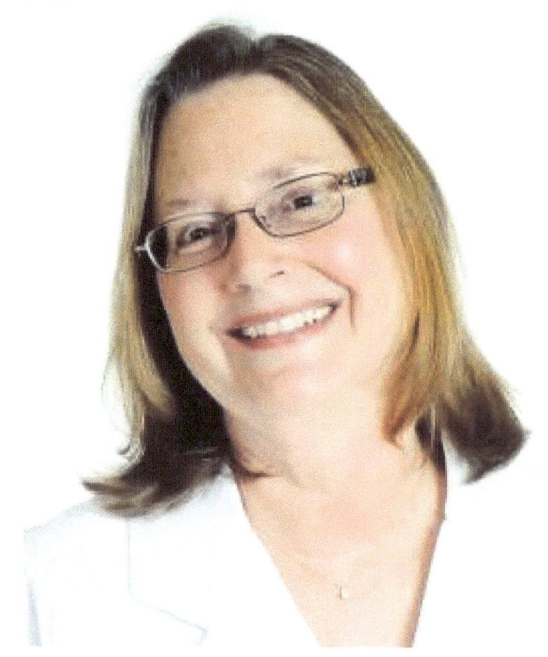

News & Views

Earlier this month, I put out a forward-facing announcement about the issue of HOPE Magazine that you've just read. In that announcement, I shared that stories in this issue would be among some of the rawest that we've published to date.

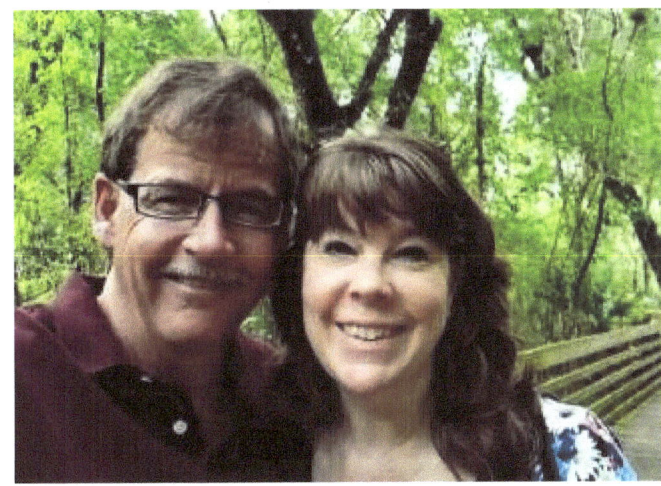

As I write this closing note today, I just completed the final layout of the magazine. While every story touches me deeply, several of this month's stories moved me to tears. As a father who raised four sons, Bode's story really touched my heart. That old saying that *'life is what happens when you are making other plans'* is such a truth.

One of our stories had to be edited significantly prior to publication. In the initial email to me, the author noted that there were many PTSD triggers in his life's story. Mindful of our readership, the harshest-of-the-harsh points needed to be edited out, though we went to great lengths to honor his story – and his life.

Every single contributor has shared stories of courage and inspiration. Most will never make the evening news, but such is the nature of those who choose to put their life's experience out there to serve a greater good. They lift humanity higher.

To all our contributors who, since our 2013 launch, have had the courage to share their stories, we thank you. For those yet to share, perhaps it's time. You can be part of helping light the path for those who need it most – brain injury survivors and those who love them.

Peace,

~ David & Sarah

www.ingramcontent.com/pod-product-compliance
Lightning Source LLC
Chambersburg PA
CBHW060811290526

45792CB00005BA/1611